The Weight Is Over

Your Guide To A Slimmer You

FRANCISCA M. JOHNSON

TABLE OF CONTENTS

Acknowledgement
Dedication
Introduction: My Weight Struggle

CHAPTER 1.. 1
CHAPTER 2.. 6
CHAPTER 3... 15
CHAPTER 4... 24
CHAPTER 5... 33
CHAPTER 6... 44
CONCLUSION...61

ACKNOWLEDGEMENT

This journey has been an aggregate undertaking, and I'm profoundly thankful for the embroidery of help and motivation that has molded my way to a better life.

To my family, whose affection and consolation have been the bedrock of my excursion. Your faithful help pushed me forward when the street was testing, and for that, I am significantly appreciative.

To my companions, who gave a shout out to me and praised every little triumph. Your faith in me was a consistent update that I was never alone on this mission.

To the specialists and experts who imparted their insight and directed me to shrewdness, I owe you an obligation of appreciation. Your bits of knowledge were guides on the way to a better life.

To the numerous people who shared their own accounts, battles, and wins, you advised me that this journey is a common one, and I'm enlivened by your solidarity and versatility.

This affirmation is a demonstration of the force of the local area and shared encounters chasing a better life. Much thanks to you for being a part of this fantastic experience.

DEDICATION

In my quest for better days, I discovered my inner explorer,
A spirit that refused to surrender,
A soul in pursuit of greater well-being,
This narrative is our story.

To my beloved family and friends,
Your support was my anchor.
You illuminated my path and whispered words of encouragement.
Through your love, I found strength.

To the trials that dotted my path,
You were not adversaries but mentors,
Every stumble is a lesson.
Guiding me on this quest to a healthier life

In the quiet of the evening, as I savored my journey,
I found beauty in each moment.
And etched lessons deep into my heart,
This is not just my story; it's ours.

INTRODUCTION

MY WEIGHT STRUGGLE

Life frequently gives us challenges that characterize the course of our excursion and rouse us to set out on groundbreaking journeys. As far as I'm concerned, quite possibly the most significant test I've confronted has been the determined fight with abundant weight. A fight reverberates with many—a battle that can feel like a ceaseless move up a precarious mountain.

The underlying foundations of my weight reduction venture trace back to an essential second in my life—a second when I could never again overlook the gravity of my weight issue and its unavoidable effect on my wellbeing, confidence, and, generally speaking, prosperity. This second turned into a source of inspiration, an enlivening that I was unable to excuse any more. It constrained me to stand up to not just the actual changes I expected to make but also the inward ones, underscoring that the way to weight reduction isn't just about shedding pounds; it's tied in with rediscovering oneself, encouraging self-esteem, and embracing a better, more joyful presence.

In the chapters that follow, I welcome you to go along with me on a profoundly private journey of self-revelation, flexibility, and change. This record isn't solely about weight loss; it's a show of the vigor of the human spirit, the meaning of certainty, and the mission for a predominant interpretation of oneself. Along the way, I encountered wins and misfortunes, epiphanies, and uncertainty; however, above all,I uncovered a recharged feeling of direction and enduring assurance. Together, how about we set out on this adventure? The weight is over, and now is the right time to embrace the better, more joyful you that is standing by.

CHAPTER 1

THE TURNING POINT

In life, every journey of transformation has a pivotal moment—an instant when the world we've known tilts and we find ourselves standing at a crossroads. This chapter, my turning point, addresses the end of long periods of battle, self-question, and the evident acknowledgment that I could never again bear the weight, both physical and profound, that had held me in its grasp for a really long time.

The Breaking Moment: Acknowledging My Weight Struggle

The roots of my weight loss journey extend deep into my past, threading through countless moments of inner turmoil, anxiety, and, at times, self-loathing. Yet, it was a single-breaking moment that would set the stage for the journey that was about to unfold.

The breaking point was an unforgiving reflection in the mirror, one that I could no longer avoid. It was an image that was harsh and unrelenting—an image I could no longer pretend didn't exist. I stood before my own reflection, and there it was—the embodiment of the struggle that had become my daily companion—excess weight.

The mirror did not lie; it revealed the extra pounds that had encroached upon my body, the weight that had surreptitiously crept into my life, steadily and persistently. There was a visible impact on my health, both physically and emotionally.

The breaking moment was something other than a visual experience. It was a significant acknowledgment of the unmistakable cost that excess weight was taking on my life. I was wrestling with an expanding weight issue, one that was testing my day-to-day exercises, my energy levels, and my general prosperity. It was no longer something I could overlook or hide where no one would think to look; it had developed into a squeezing worry that requested consideration.

The mirror not only mirrored the actual impacts of my weight battle but additionally uncovered the effect on my confidence and fearlessness. It was unsettling to observe the individual in the reflection who appeared so far from the picture I held of me. The breaking moment was not just about the truth of my actual appearance; it was about the disintegration of my confidence, the quiet cost taken on by my self-esteem, and the manner in which it impacted my communications with the world.

The profound weight was becoming as oppressive as the actual pounds. It was the uncertainty, the distress, and the interior scrutiny that played mind-numbingly repetitive to me. I scrutinized my value, my capacity, and my entitlement to feel certain about my own skin. The breaking moment was not only a visual retribution; it was a close-to-home retribution as well.

My journey toward a better, more joyful me started with this breaking moment, a second that requested affirmation and prodded me to face what was happening. It was a snapshot of retribution with the truth of my weight, a snapshot of acknowledgment, and, at last, a second that implied a source of inspiration.

A Crossroad: The Decision to Change

The breaking moment was an impetus for change, yet it was only the start. It denoted the second when I ended up remaining at a junction, confronted with decisions that would decide the heading of my excursion. I was keenly conscious that I could decide to go on down the natural way, notwithstanding its distress and the feeling of being caught. It was a way I had realized well, one that was characterized by the state of affairs, a way I had followed for a really long time.

It was the way of idleness, where change was stayed away from, and the recognizable, however awkward, gave a feeling of safety. On the other hand, there was the way more uncommon, the one that guaranteed change. It was the way I had thought about it, however, never sincerely sought after. This way, I addressed a jump into the obscure, a readiness to embrace change, and a guarantee of defying the obstructions that had kept me down.

As I remained at this junction, I perceived the meaning of the decision before me. I knew that the choice to set out on the excursion of change was not to be trifled with. It was a choice that required assurance, responsibility, and strength. It was a promise to oneself, a statement that my prosperity and self-esteem had the right to become the overwhelming focus.

The choice to change was an act of pure trust, an eagerness to break free from the shackles of carelessness, and a statement that I was prepared to recover command over my life. It was not just about shedding the excess pounds; it was tied in with unburdening myself from the weight that had held me hostage in different parts of my life.

Finding Purpose: Discovering My 'Why'

As I ventured further into my weight-loss journey, I discovered a profound sense of purpose. It was more than just the desire to look better in clothes or reach a particular number on the scale. My purpose was rooted in a deep yearning to improve my health, to nurture my self-worth, and to seize the opportunity to lead a healthier, happier life.

This purpose became my 'why,' the driving force behind my commitment to change. It was the reason I chose the path of transformation at the crossroads, and it remained the motivation that propelled me forward. My 'why' became the anchor that kept me rooted during moments of doubt and the torch that illuminated the path ahead.

My journey was no longer just about shedding pounds; it was about finding my way back to self-love and self-acceptance. It was about rewriting the script that had been playing in my mind, one filled with self-doubt and criticism. It was about embracing a renewed sense of self-worth and confidence, understanding that I deserved to live my life to the fullest.

This chapter, The Turning Point, is the inception of my quest for a healthier, happier existence. It symbolizes the beginning of a journey that was marked by both challenges and victories, moments of clarity and doubt, and above all, the unwavering determination to overcome my weight struggle and claim a better, brighter future. In the following chapters, I will delve deeper into the science of transformation, the steps I took to make progress, and the mindset shifts that paved the way for success. This journey is not just about my transformation; it's about the collective strength we possess to overcome obstacles and redefine our lives. It's a reminder that weight is more than numbers on a scale; it signifies the reclamation of life and the discovery of the extraordinary potential that lies within each one of us.

CHAPTER 2

THE SCIENCE OF TRANSFORMATION

In the past chapter, we dove into my own journey's beginning, set apart by a critical defining moment. It was a second that constrained me to recognize my weight battle, to confront the obvious truth of overabundance pounds, and to go with the significant choice to change. This chapter, Chapter 2, will take us more deeply into the journey and investigate the science behind change. It's a journey set apart by flexibility, assurance, and the quest for a better, more joyful me.

Understanding the Battle: The Science Behind Weight Loss

To embark on the journey of transformation, one must first grasp the scientific principles that underpin the battle with weight. It's essential to comprehend the intricacies of how the body stores and expends energy and, most importantly, the mechanics of weight gain and weight loss.

Our bodies are incredibly efficient machines. They utilize food as fuel, extracting energy from the nutrients we consume, particularly carbohydrates, fats, and proteins. This energy is essential for everyday functions, from basic bodily functions such as breathing and digesting to more active pursuits like walking, running, and even thinking.

The energy balance equation is the cornerstone of weight management. In essence, it signifies that the energy we consume (in the form of food) should be balanced with the energy we expend (through daily activities and exercise). If we consume more energy than we burn, the surplus is stored as fat, leading to weight gain. Conversely, if we expend more energy than we consume, our bodies tap into stored fat for energy, leading to weight loss.

The challenge of weight loss is intricately connected to the balance of calorie intake and expenditure. To effectively shed pounds, one must create a calorie deficit by either consuming fewer calories, expending more through exercise, or a combination of both. The core principle is simple, yet the application can be complex.

Understanding the science of weight loss also involves recognizing the role of metabolism. Metabolism is the body's engine for energy expenditure, and it's influenced by factors such as age, gender, genetics, and muscle mass. In this regard, muscle plays a vital role. Muscle tissue is metabolically active, meaning it burns more calories at rest compared to fat. Hence, building and maintaining muscle is essential for a more efficient metabolism.

Weight loss isn't solely about reducing fat; it's also about preserving lean muscle. When the body loses weight, it doesn't exclusively shed fat. Lean muscle may also be affected, and this is a critical consideration. The loss of muscle can negatively impact metabolism, making it more challenging to maintain weight loss.

Furthermore, the science of weight loss is significantly intertwined with hormones. Hormones regulate a myriad of processes in the body, including hunger, satiety, and the way our bodies store and use fat. Ghrelin, often referred to as the "hunger hormone," stimulates appetite, while leptin, the "satiety hormone," conveys a sense of fullness.

In overweight or obese individuals, hormonal imbalances can disrupt these signals. This can lead to persistent feelings of hunger and reduced satisfaction after eating. Weight loss can help to correct these imbalances, making it easier to control appetite and manage portion sizes.

Perhaps the most basic chemical connected with weight reduction is insulin. Insulin is created by the pancreas and is responsible for directing glucose levels. At the point when we consume carbs, our bodies separate them into glucose, which enters the circulatory system. Insulin then works with the take-up of glucose by our cells, where it's utilized for energy. Any excess glucose is put away in the liver and muscles as glycogen. Assuming these stockpiling regions are full, excess glucose is converted into fat.

Insulin's role in weighing the executives is critical. In conditions like insulin resistance, a condition seen as often as possible in overweight or stout people, the body's cells become less receptive to insulin. This prompts higher insulin levels, which can increase the capacity of the body to store glucose as fat.

Weight reduction procedures frequently include measures to further develop insulin awareness, like diminishing carb consumption and expanding active work. This can bring about better glucose control and more productive fat usage.

Vitally, the study of change requires a comprehension of the intricacies of fat cells. Fat tissue, regularly alluded to as fat, assumes a complex role in the body. It has the capability to hold energy and secrete chemicals, for example, adiponectin and leptin, that impact digestion and craving.

Furthermore, fat cells are sorted into two kinds: white fat tissue and brown fat tissue. White fat essentially fills in as energy stockpiling, while earthy-colored fat is engaged with heat creation. Actuating earthy-colored fat might possibly increase calorie use, adding to weight reduction.

Understanding the science behind weight loss looks like deciphering the body's secret code. It requires grasping the amicability between calorie affirmation and use, the occupation of assimilation, the impact of synthetic substances, and the intricacies of fat cells. Armed with this data, we can tailor our techniques and approaches for convincing, sensible weight loss.

Setting the Course: Defining My Weight Loss Goals

The foundation of a successful weight loss journey is the establishment of clear, achievable goals. Goals provide direction, motivation, and a yardstick for measuring progress. They transform our desire for change into tangible, actionable steps.

In defining my weight loss goals, I embarked on a journey of self-reflection. What did I want to achieve, and what was the timeline for my transformation? Setting specific, measurable, and realistic goals was paramount. Rather than a vague desire to "lose weight," I decided on a target number of pounds to shed, a realistic timeframe, and the commitment to make steady, sustainable progress.

Additionally, it was essential to consider non-scale victories. Weight loss is about more than numbers on a scale; it's about feeling healthier, experiencing increased energy, and regaining self-confidence. These non-scale victories became an integral part of my goals.

Moreover, I aimed to break my long-term goals into smaller, manageable milestones. These short-term goals offered a sense of achievement and helped maintain motivation on the journey.

In this chapter, we've explored the science behind weight loss, delving into the calorie balance equation, metabolism, hormonal regulation, and the intricacies of fat cells. We've also recognized the significance of setting clear, achievable goals as the initial step towards effective and sustainable weight loss.

Our journey has only just begun, and in the upcoming chapters, we will delve deeper into the practical steps I took to put the science into action. From managing diet and portion control to incorporating exercise and cultivating mindful eating habits, these chapters will shed light on the practical strategies that marked my path towards transformation.

The wisdom of weight loss has laid the foundation, but the true metamorphosis lies in the operation of this knowledge. Together, let's unravel the complications of metamorphosis and uncover the strategies that can help you achieve your weight loss goals.

Planning for Success: Crafting My Strategy

With a grasp of the science behind weight loss and well-defined goals, the next step on my journey was to craft a strategy that would guide my path to transformation. Success in weight loss, as with any endeavor, requires a well-thought-out plan, a roadmap that provides direction and structure.

The key components of a successful weight loss strategy include dietary choices, exercise routines, and the cultivation of mindful eating habits. Let's delve into each of these facets:

Dietary Choices: The Foundation of Weight Loss

Diet assumes a certain part in the weight reduction venture. It's the foundation upon which viable and feasible weight reduction is constructed. My dietary decisions turned into an essential part of my methodology, zeroing in on making better, more cognizant choices about the food sources I ate.

One of the most vital phases in my process was to lay out a calorie shortage, where I consumed fewer calories than I exhausted. Accomplishing this shortage frequently implies diminishing part estimates, picking supplement-rich food varieties, and rehearsing balance. I perceived that it wasn't necessary to focus on denying myself yet about going with smart decisions.

One more essential part of my dietary system was the decrease in handled and high-sugar food varieties. These things frequently contain void calories and contribute to changes in glucose levels, which can prompt expanded appetites and desires. By focusing on entire food sources, natural products, vegetables, lean proteins, and solid fats, I guaranteed that my body got the fundamental supplements for supported energy and prosperity.

Moreover, hydration was the foundation of my dietary technique. Drinking a sufficient amount of water upholds general wellbeing and helps control hunger. Remaining very hydrated can lessen the probability of mistaking hunger for hunger, finally forestalling pointless calorie utilization.

In making a fruitful dietary system, I found the meaning of dinner arranging. Getting ready for dinners ahead of time saved me and empowered me to pursue better decisions. It forestalled imprudent, less nutritious choices and permitted me to control segment sizes.

Exercise Routines: The Key to Sustainable Weight Loss

Integrating exercise into my day-to-day schedule was a critical part of my weight reduction procedure. Active work assumes a fundamental role in both weight reduction and, generally speaking, wellbeing. It assists with reducing the calorie deficit required for weight reduction and advances cardiovascular wellbeing, muscle advancement, and further developed digestion.

My workout routine was not about outrageous exercises but rather about consistency. I began with exercises I delighted in, like energetic strolling, swimming, or cycling. Bit by bit, I expanded the power and span of my exercises as my wellness level moved along.

Cardiovascular activities, such as running or cycling, were vital for consuming calories and further developing heart wellbeing. Moreover, strength-building exercises like weightlifting or bodyweight exercises have become an indispensable piece of my daily practice. These activities assisted form and safeguard with inclining bulk, supporting a more proficient digestion.

The way to improve outcomes in practice was to find exercises I delighted in and make them a normal part of my life. I observed that consistency was definitely more powerful than inconsistent, focused energy exercises that could prompt burnout. By integrating active work into my day-to-day routine, it turned into a maintainable, long-term propensity.

Cultivating Mindful Eating Habits: Nourishing Body and Soul

Careful eating turned into the last piece of my methodology for effective weight reduction. It's tied in with being available and mindful during dinners, appreciating each nibble, and figuring out the signs of yearning and totality that our bodies give.

Perhaps the most groundbreaking practice I took on was eating gradually. This permitted me to relish the flavors and surfaces of my food, yet it also permitted my body to convey messages of completion prior to indulging.

Portion control is one more fundamental part of careful eating. I figured out how to perceive fitting part measures and to keep away from the normal propensity for "cleaning the plate" in any event, when I felt full.

Also, careful eating included paying attention to my body's yearning prompts. It implied eating when I was ravenous and halting when I was fulfilled, as opposed to eating for profound reasons or without really thinking.

To work with careful eating, I limited interruptions during dinners, for example, sitting in front of the TV or utilizing my cell phone. All things considered, I zeroed in on the demonstration of eating and partaking in my food.

The act of careful eating not only assisted me with pursuing more cognizant food decisions but additionally encouraged a better relationship with food. It permitted me to see the value in the supporting and pleasurable parts of eating while at the same time diminishing profound and careless eating.

In this chapter, we've revealed the basic components of creating an effective weight reduction system. Dietary decisions, workout schedules, and the development of careful dietary patterns all play an essential role in achieving compelling and maintainable weight reduction. Every viewpoint is interconnected, shaping an extensive way to deal with change.

As we proceed with our journey, these components will be coordinated into a useful aide for executing the systems that prompted my effective weight reduction. Through a mix of science, arranging, and care, we'll reveal the way to a better, more joyful you.

In the ensuing parts, we'll investigate the useful parts of my excursion, including dietary changes, portion control, workout schedules, and the improvement of careful dietary patterns. This complex methodology will uncover how I applied the logical standards examined in this part to accomplish a successful and reasonable weight reduction.

CHAPTER 3

PROGRESS IN ACTION

Welcome to chapter 3 of our journey, where we shift our concentration to the reasonable parts of changing our lives. We've proactively investigated the basic science behind weight reduction and fostered a complete methodology for progress. Presently, now is the right time to set that methodology in motion.

A New Way of Eating: Tackling My Dietary Habits

Dietary propensities assume a vital role in our weight reduction venture. While the science behind weight reduction gives important experiences, our everyday food decisions make an interpretation of hypotheses into results.

My journey towards a better, more joyful me started with a profound jump into my dietary propensities. I perceived that for practical weight reduction, I expected to develop a better relationship with food. This didn't mean totally taking out the food sources I adored; rather, it included making informed decisions and fostering a careful way to deal with eating.

We should investigate a portion of the key dietary changes that became necessary to my change:

1. Emphasizing Nutrient-Dense Foods

One of the foundations of my better approach to eating was focusing on supplement-rich food sources. These are food sources that are plentiful in fundamental supplements, including nutrients, minerals, and cancer prevention agents, while being moderately low in calories. Consider mixed greens, vivid vegetables, lean proteins, entire grains, and healthy fats.

By integrating these food varieties into my everyday dinners, I guaranteed that my body got the essential supplements for ideal working. Supplement-rich food sources support general wellbeing as well as assist in making a sensation of completion, which with canning check gorging.

2. Reducing Processed Foods

Processed foods, often loaded with additives, preservatives, and excess sugars, became a target for reduction in my dietary overhaul. These foods are often calorie-dense and nutrient-poor, making it easy to consume excessive calories without feeling satisfied.

Minimizing processed foods meant reading labels and opting for whole, unprocessed alternatives. It was about choosing whole grains over refined grains, whole fruits over fruit juices, and whole ingredients over artificial additives.

3. Managing Carbohydrate Intake

Sugars are a wellspring of energy for the body; however, not all carbs are made equal. I embraced a fair way to deal with carbs, zeroing in on complex carbs that give supported energy and advance completion. These included food varieties like entire grains, vegetables, and bland vegetables.

I additionally became aware of added sugars, perceiving that overabundance sugar can prompt spikes in glucose levels and ensuing accidents, setting off appetite and desires. This implies restricting sweet bites, improved drinks, and treats.

4. Incorporating Healthy Fats

In opposition to the fantasy that fat ought to be avoided, I discovered that healthy fats are fundamental to my prosperity. Avocado, nuts, seeds, and olive oil became ordinary parts of my eating regimen. These solid fats provided satiety as well as upheld essential physical processes, including the ingestion of fat-solvent nutrients.

5. Practicing Portion Control

Portion control was a distinct advantage in my weight reduction venture. It permitted me to partake in the food varieties I cherished without indulging. I began utilizing more modest plates and utensils, which normally restricted segment sizes. This straightforward change made it simpler to try not to consume excessive calories.

I additionally turned out to be more aware of serving sizes while feasting out. It wasn't necessary to focus on denying myself, however, enjoying the kinds of sensible pieces. By eating gradually and focusing on my body's appetite prompts, I guaranteed that I felt fulfilled without gorging.

These dietary changes shaped the underpinnings of my better approach to eating. It wasn't actually necessary to focus on unbending limitations or hardship; it was tied in with pursuing informed decisions and focusing on food varieties that supported both my body and my soul.

Portion Control: Managing My Appetite

Portion control is an amazing asset in the domain of weight reduction. It's tied in with grasping the size of servings and directing food consumption. This approach permits you to partake in your #1 food sources without the culpability that frequently goes with overindulgence.

The idea of portion control was indispensable to my journey, as it gave me a pragmatic and supportable method for dealing with my cravings and calorie consumption. Here are a few systems that assisted me in becoming the best at segment control:

1. Smaller Plates and Utensils

One of the best and most straightforward strategies for segment control is utilizing more modest plates and utensils. Research shows that we will more often than not eat bigger portions when we serve ourselves on bigger plates, as it outwardly creates the impression that we're not getting sufficient food on more modest plates. By scaling back your dinnerware, you normally reduce portion sizes.

2. Be Mindful of Restaurant Portions

While eating out, it's normal for eateries to serve bigger portions than we really need. To battle this, I fostered a propensity for imparting dishes to a companion or promptly mentioning a to-go compartment for half of my dinner. This assisted with portion control as well as giving a heavenly extra dinner the following day.

3. Listen to Your Body

Your body is, in many cases, the best sign of when you've had enough to eat. By focusing on your body's appetite and totality prompts, you can abstain from indulging. Eat gradually, appreciate each chomp, and respite between nibbles to evaluate your degree of completion. This training permits your body to flag when it's fulfilled.

4. Pre-Portion Snacks

Eating can be a trap with regards to portion control. To try not to carelessly crunch on snacks directly from the sack, I started pre-portioning them into little compartments or nibbling estimated baggies. This approach made it more straightforward to partake in a wonderful nibble without overindulging.

5. Careful Eating Practices

Careful eating was an extraordinary part of my excursion towards segment control. This approach includes being completely present during dinners, enjoying each chomp, and focusing on the tactile experience of eating. By rehearsing care, I developed a more profound association with the food I devoured.

This is the way I integrated careful eating into my daily schedule:

- **Eating without Interruptions**: I tried to appreciate dinners without interruptions like the TV, PC, or cell phone. By

- zeroing in exclusively on the demonstration of eating, I could relish the flavors and surfaces of the food.
- **Biting Completely**: Biting each chomp completely helps processing as well as permits you to perceive when you're full. It requires investment for your body to convey messages of completion to your mind at such a leisurely pace, and pondering biting can assist with forestalling gorging.
- **Partaking in the Occasion**: I paused for a minute before every feast to see the value in the sustenance and joy that food brings. This training made a more certain relationship with eating.
- **Paying Attention to Yearning Signals**: By paying attention to my body's appetite prompts, I figured out how to recognize actual yearning and profound desires. This permitted me to eat when I was truly ravenous and stop when I was fulfilled.

A Journey to Exercise: Getting Active

While dietary decisions and part control are central parts of weight reduction, actual work is similarly urgent. Practice helps with calorie deficiency as well as offers a horde of medical advantages, from cardiovascular wellbeing to muscle improvement and digestion support.

My journey to a more dynamic way of life was set apart by the acknowledgment that exercise wasn't exclusively about serious exercises or rebuffing systems. All things considered, it was tied to finding exercises I delighted in and making them a standard part of my life.

We should investigate how I integrated practice into my day-to-day daily schedule:

1. Finding Enjoyable Exercises

Practice turned into a delight when I found exercises that impacted me. I investigated various choices, from energetic strolling and cycling to swimming and moving. The key was to track down exercises that I anticipated, making exercise something I truly appreciated.

2. Steady Movement

I understood that consistency was more significant than force. As opposed to beginning with arduous exercises, I started with moderate activity that lined up with my wellness level. As my perseverance and strength improved, I step-by-step expanded the force and span of my exercises.

3. Cardiovascular Activities

Cardiovascular activities, like running, cycling, and swimming, assumed a critical role in my weight reduction venture. These exercises consumed calories as well as further developed my heart's wellbeing and perseverance. A couple of meetings of cardiovascular activity each week added to my calorie consumption.

4. Strength Training

Strength training workouts, which included utilizing loads or one's body weight, were integrated to assemble and keep up with bulk. Muscle is metabolically dynamic, meaning it consumes a greater number of calories than fat. By expanding my bulk, I achieved more effective digestion.

5. Adaptability and Balance

Notwithstanding cardiovascular and strength training, I perceived the significance of adaptability and balance. Yoga and extending schedules worked on my adaptability, lessened the risk of injury, and, generally speaking, promoted actual prosperity.

6. Consistency Over Force

The key to my workout routine was consistency. Rather than irregular, focused energy exercises that could prompt burnout, I focused on normal, actual work. This approach made practice a reasonable propensity as well as worked on my general wellness.

By consolidating these activity methodologies, I integrated actual work into my everyday existence. It turned into a piece of my daily practice, much the same as cleaning my teeth or having dinner. This approach added to my weight reduction as well as worked on my general wellbeing and prosperity.

In this chapter, we've investigated the functional parts of our weight reduction venture. We've figured out how to settle on informed dietary decisions, ace piece control, and embrace active work as a cheerful piece of our lives. The combination of these techniques makes you one step closer to a better, more joyful you.

As we proceed with our excursion, we'll dive further into the outlook shifts and close-to-home viewpoints that assume an urgent role in supportable weight reduction. It's not just about changing our bodies; it's tied in with changing our relationship with food, exercise, and ourselves. Together, we'll reveal the all-encompassing way to deal with weight reduction that goes beyond numbers on a scale, cultivating confidence, strength, and enduring change.

In the forthcoming chapters, we'll investigate the close-to-home and mental aspects of weight reduction, grasp the significance of emotionally supportive networks, and praise the triumphs en route. Weight reduction isn't simply a physical journey; it's a change of mind, body, and soul.

CHAPTER 4

A MINDFUL SHIFT

In this section, we'll investigate the force of a careful shift on our weight reduction venture. This shift includes a significant impact in context, embracing care in each part of our change.

Embracing Mindful Eating: A New Approach

As I progressed forward with my journey to a better me, I coincidentally found a progressive methodology that fundamentally altered the manner in which I connected with food—careful eating. This wasn't simply one more eating routine or weight reduction trend; it was a significant change in my way of dealing with supporting my body.

Everything began with relishing each chomp. I understood that for quite a long time, I had been eating carelessly, hurrying through dinners, or eating down food while working or staring at the television. Be that as it may, with careful eating, I figured out how to dial back and genuinely experience the flavors, surfaces, and smells of every piece.

Imagine enjoying a strawberry as though it were the very first you'd tasted. The delicious eruption of flavor, the difference between pleasantness and tartness—it was a disclosure. I ended up savoring even the most straightforward dinners as though they were connoisseur feasts.

Paying attention to my body has become my core value. Before each feast, I'd stop and ask myself, "Am I really ravenous, or am I eating without much forethought?" It was a groundbreaking inquiry. I started to comprehend that my body had its own particular way of letting me know when it required sustenance.

During meals, I'd check in with my body's signs. I didn't simply thoughtlessly complete everything on my plate; I ate until I was satisfied. Furthermore, learn to expect the unexpected. I frequently found that I didn't require as much food as I remembered to feel content. It was a disclosure—careful eating was assisting me with lessening indulging.

Breaking free from profound eating was a difficult yet fundamental piece of this new methodology. Food had been my solace in the midst of stress, trouble, or weariness. Be that as it may, presently, I am figuring out how to recognize my feelings without going to food as a prop.

At the point when feelings emerged, I'd respite and take a full breath. I'd ask myself, "Am I eating since I'm eager or on the grounds that I'm feeling a specific way?" There wasn't really any need to focus on denying my sentiments, yet I tend to express them in a better manner. I'd take a walk, practice profound breathing, or just sit with my feelings without going after a bite.

Rehearsing careful eating includes useful advances. I set up for every dinner, establishing a tranquil climate without interruptions. I switched off the television and set aside my telephone. I even lit a light every so often, transforming supper time into something somewhat customary.

I bit my food gradually, appreciating each chomp. The surface, the taste—maybe I was finding the delight of eating once more. I connected with my faculties, appreciating the visual allure and smell of my food. I offered thanks for the sustenance my dinner provided.

It wasn't really necessary to focus on unbending standards or denying myself treats. I let myself appreciate desires without judgment, for however long they were, with some restraint. Careful nibbling turned into a propensity as well. I pre-parceled my tidbits and stayed away from careless chomping.

Embracing mindful eating resembles setting out on a journey of self-disclosure. It was tied in with sustaining my body, paying attention to its requirements, and cultivating a positive relationship with food. With each careful nibble, I felt more on top of my body, and the excursion to a better me became an actual change as well as a profoundly private one.

Breaking Through Plateaus: Overcoming Challenges

As I advanced on my weight reduction venture, I experienced a typical hindrance that many face: plateaus. These times of obvious stagnation can be dispiriting, yet they can likewise act as open doors for development and change.

The Frustration of Plateaus

It is frustrating to hit a plateau. You've been diligently following your eating regimen and working out every day, seeing consistent improvement, and then, unexpectedly, it seems like you've run into a stopping point. The numbers on the scale will not move, and it's not difficult to feel deterred.

Understanding Plateaus

To overcome plateaus, it's fundamental to first figure them out. Plateaus regularly happen for a couple of reasons:

- **Metabolic Variation**: Your body adjusts to your new eating regimen and work-out daily schedule, which can dial back weight reduction.
- **Water Maintenance**: Your body might hold water, concealing fat misfortune on the scale.
- **Loss of Muscle**: Quick weight reduction can bring about the deficiency of fit bulk, which can dial back your digestion.
- **Hormonal Changes**: Hormonal shifts, particularly in women, can influence weight reduction progress.

Strategies to Break Through Plateaus

Plateaus might appear to be unconquerable, yet with the right strategies, they can be survived. This is the way I explored these difficulties:

1. Change Your Caloric Intake

At the point when your body adjusts to your ongoing calorie consumption, now is the ideal time to adapt. Somewhat decreasing your everyday calories or changing your macronutrient proportions can launch your digestion.

2. Fluctuate Your Exercises

Variety in your workout routine keeps your body from adjusting. Attempt various sorts of exercises, integrate strength training, and increase the power to keep your digestion dynamic.

3. Monitor Your Stress Levels

Stress can increase plateaus. Track down pressure-decrease methods that work for you, like contemplation, yoga, or profound breathing activities. Bringing down feelings of anxiety can support weight reduction.

4. Remain Hydrated

Satisfactory hydration is vital for maintaining sound digestion. Drinking sufficient water can assist with decreasing water maintenance and boosting overall wellbeing.

5. Get Adequate Rest

Quality rest assumes a critical role in weight reduction. Hold back nothing for long stretches of rest each evening. Inadequate rest can disrupt hormonal equilibrium and slow down your digestion.

6. Be Patient and Tireless

Plateaus are important for the journey. It's vital to remain patient and tireless. Celebrate non-scale triumphs, for example, expanded energy levels or further developed wellness, to remain spurred.

7. Look for Help

Some of the time, getting through a plateau might need the help and direction of a medical services professional or an enrolled dietitian. Make it a point to seek master counsel when required.

My Personal Plateau Breakthrough

I distinctively recall the plateau I experienced on my journey. It seemed like I was stuck for quite a long time, and it was demoralizing. In any case, I advised myself that plateaus are a characteristic piece of the cycle.

I chose to change my caloric intake and my meals. I likewise consolidated extreme cardio exercise into my workout schedule. It was intense right away; however, the progression paid off. I got through the plateau; however, I likewise felt more animated and grounded than any other time in recent memory.

Getting through a plateau showed me the value of flexibility and persistence on this journey. It's not just about the objective; it's about the examples advanced en route. Each test, including plateaus, is a chance for development and change. By grasping the explanations for plateaus and executing the right procedures, you can keep advancing on your way to a better you.

Finding Support: Staying Motivated

On the twisting road to weight reduction, there are times when the journey feels like an independent undertaking. However, it's during those snapshots of isolation that the force of help turns out to be

generally obvious. Finding the right emotionally supportive network can revive your inspiration and keep the fires of your weight reduction objectives burning brilliantly.

The Solitary Journey

Weight reduction can at times feel like a solitary journey, with the heaviness of your objectives laying exclusively on your shoulders. In those minutes, it's not difficult to become dispirited, and self-uncertainty can begin to sneak in. It's the point at which we really want some assistance or a cordial face the most.

The Power of Support

Support isn't simply a pleasant thing to have; it's a distinct advantage. Whether it's family, companions, a care group, or a web-based local area, the force of help lies in its capacity to lift you up when you want it most. An update: You're in good company on your journey.

Loved Ones

Your prompt circle can be an inconceivable wellspring of inspiration. Share your objectives with your friends and family, and you may be astounded at how they rally behind you. They can offer support and understanding, and now and again, they might actually go along with you on your journey.

Accountability Partners

Having an accountability partner can be a strong inspiration. This can be a companion who shares your objectives or an expert like a

fitness coach or an enlisted dietitian. They can assist you with keeping focused, praise your victories, and give direction when you face difficulties.

Support Gatherings

Support gatherings and online networks offer an extraordinary type of association. In these spaces, you'll find people who personally comprehend the promising and less promising times of the weight reduction venture. They offer a place of refuge to share your encounters, look for exhortation, and draw motivation from the triumphs of others.

The Power of Shared Goals

At the point when you're encircled by individuals who share your objectives, something unimaginable occurs. You draw inspiration from each other, celebrating your singular triumphs as well as the aggregate advancement of your gathering. Shared objectives create a sense of brotherhood and a common perspective.

My Support System

On my journey, I found the unfathomable worth of help. My loved ones energized behind me, offering support and a listening ear when I really wanted it most. My exercise mate turned into my accomplice in the works, and we pushed each other higher than ever.

I likewise found a strong web-based local area where I could share my encounters, gain from others, and give direction as a trade-off. It was a help on the harder days, an update that I was essential for an option that could be greater than simply my own journey.

Keep in mind that the weight reduction venture doesn't need to be a singular undertaking. Search out the help you really want, whether from friends and family, experts, or similar people. In these associations, you'll track down the inspiration to continue to push ahead, in any event, when the way forward feels testing. Embrace the force of help, and let it fuel your passion to arrive at your objectives.

CHAPTER 5

THE LONG-TERM VIEW

In my journey to practical weight loss, I showed up with a huge comprehension: the somewhat long view truly matters. A perspective transcends the appeal of helpful arrangements, crash diets, and quick results. It's connected to embracing the outing as a tremendous change, mentioning determination, obligation, and an adjustment of mindset.

The Trickiness of Helpful Arrangements

Our world is doused with responsibilities for transient weight loss plans. It's the 30-day challenge, the detox purge, and the charmed pill that seem to offer quick results. In any case, through my trip, I've found that these substitute ways habitually lead to frustration. They could make short-lived changes, yet they only, from time to time, convey the perseverance through change we search for. The excessively long view assists us with seeing past these misdirections and embracing them in a more sensible manner.

Grasping the Long-Term View

The long-term view starts with an adjustment of settings. Seeing weight decrease isn't solely about showing up at a captivated number on the scale. It's a journey into self-disclosure, self-improvement, and certainty. Permit me to take you through the central guidelines of this noteworthy methodology.

1. Resilience as an Uprightness

Resilience transforms into the underpinning of your outing. In a world acquainted with second fulfillment, steadiness is an uprightness that can be attempted to create. The fact that enduring change requires venture makes, in any case, it apparent. Through my experiences, I've come to see the value of steadiness, despite weight loss targets.

2. The Impact of Consistency

Consistency is where authentic charm happens. It's about those everyday affinities and choices that, over an extended period of time, have yielded results. My interaction showed me the importance of consistency, the power of little everyday changes, and the total impact they have on our lives.

3. Characterizing Functional Goals

Making reachable, commonsense goals is crucial eventually. It's to make some separation from setting over-the-top, unthinkable targets and, actually, making objectives that are plausible as well as reasonable. I'll walk you through the specialty of goal setting, which keeps you energized without setting you up for disappointment.

4. Embracing an all-encompassing Methodology

A thorough methodology is essential, perceiving that pragmatic change includes something past eating regimen and exercise. It's connected to supporting a superior relationship with your body, regulating pressure, and empowering self-compassion. I'll show you how a sweeping methodology conveys balance and perseverance through change in your journey.

5. Tracking down Delight in the Journey

The long-term view urges you to track down bliss in the genuine journey, not just in the goal. It's connected to complimenting non-scale wins, encouraging positive self-discernment, and sorting out some way to value yourself in the meantime. I'll plunge into the adjustment of your attitude and how it can bring joy to each step of the outing.

6. The Power of Adaptability

Adaptability is your safeguard, even with setbacks and impediments. My interaction is separated by challenges, and each one has been an opportunity for improvement and learning. I'll share the meaning of adaptability and how each challenge can be a venturing stone toward transforming into a more grounded, more grounded form of yourself.

7. Another Relationship with Food

Food isn't the enemy; it's food and a wellspring of joy. The drawn-out view changes your relationship with food, from cautious eating to chasing after better choices without difficulty. I'll frame how this shift can carry amicability to your dietary examples.

8. Staying Inspired for the Significant Length

Staying motivated all through the journey can be a test. I'll surrender strategies for keeping up with your energy, finding your unique wellsprings of motivation, and investigating periods when motivation has all the earmarks of being elusive.

Your Journey Continues

As we explore the long-term view, it's a consolation to move your perspective, reconsider your goals, and embrace a momentous excursion that unfurls after some time. Certified change goes past the numbers on a scale. It's a journey into self-disclosure, self-improvement, and certainty.

The road to persevering through change may be long, yet each step conveys that you are more like a superior, more happy, and more connected with a variant of yourself. Your interaction continues, and the goal is to create an impression of the understanding and strength you've procured along the way. Embrace the drawn-out view and let it guide you toward getting through change.

Staying on Course: My Ongoing Strategy

In the multifaceted and consistently developing journey of weight reduction, one thing turns out to be completely clear: continuing through to the end is the genuine trial of responsibility. It's not just about arriving at a particular number on the scale; it's tied in with exploring the changing scene of life while protecting the better way of life you've endeavored to accomplish. In this section, we will investigate my continuous procedure for keeping up with this unimaginable change.

The weight-upkeep Challenge

Arriving at your objective weight is a momentous achievement; however, it's simply a part of the bigger story. The genuine test starts when you mean to support that weight and the sound propensities you've developed. Weight support isn't tied in with keeping afloat;

it's about reliably pushing ahead, exploring the influxes of life while watching out for your advancement.

Grasping the Continuous System

Keeping on track requires a methodology that is reasonable as well as versatile for the rhythmic movement of day-to-day existence. It's something other than whatever you eat and how you work out; it's a way of life based on the standards of consistency, equilibrium, and flexibility. We should dive into the vital components of this continuous system, as seen from the perspective of my journey.

1. Equilibrium and Balance

Keeping up with your weight is a cautious and difficult exercise. It's tied in with tracking down the balance between partaking in the food varieties you love and keeping away from overindulgence. I've taken in the craft of control, appreciating that a periodic treat isn't a misfortune but a piece of a reasonable way of life. We'll examine procedures for keeping up with this balance and making it a consistent part of your life.

2. Customary Active Work

Exercise ought to never be deserted. It's a continuous obligation to move your body in ways you appreciate and that keep you fit. My process has shown me that this responsibility doesn't falter subsequent to arriving at an objective weight; it's a deep-rooted practice. We'll dig into how to make practice an inborn piece of your regular routine.

3. Profound Flexibility

Your close-to-home prosperity assumes a huge part in weight upkeep. Life brings its share of pressure and difficulties, yet I've found that close-to-home strength is your safeguard against them. We'll investigate methods for overseeing pressure, rehearsing self-sympathy, and sustaining close-to-home versatility to adapt to the inescapable curves that life tosses in our direction.

4. Responsibility and Backing

Responsibility doesn't vanish in the wake of hitting your objective weight. It's a steady partner. Whether it's customary registrations with an accomplice, a mentor, or a strong gathering, or the utilization of the following devices and applications, remaining responsible keeps you on the right path.

5. Careful Eating Forever

Careful eating isn't simply a stage; it's a deep-rooted practice. It's tied in with proceeding to enjoy each chomp, paying attention to your body's signals, and breaking free from profound eating designs. I'll share how this training stays a focal component of my day-to-day routine, upgrading the manner in which I interface with food.

6. Remaining Informed

The universe of sustenance and wellbeing is steadily developing. Remaining informed about the most recent explorations, patterns, and advancements is essential. My process has instructed me that the quest for information is a continuous interaction, and I'll direct you on the best way to remain refreshed and informed.

7. Putting Forth New Objectives

Arriving at a particular weight isn't as far as it goes; it's a designated spot in the excursion. We'll investigate the significance of constantly testing yourself with new goals, whether they connect with wellness, nourishment, or self-awareness.

8. Observing Achievements

It is something other than a congratulatory gesture to recognize your advancement and accomplishments; it's an imperative wellspring of inspiration. I'll show how commending every achievement, regardless of how little, energizes your assurance and keeps you mindful of exactly how far you've come.

9. Adjusting to Life Changes

Life is dynamic, as is your weight-upkeep venture. We'll talk about how to adjust to changes in your day-to-day existence, whether they include vocation, family, or individual conditions, while still remaining consistent with your solid way of life.

10. The Continuous Change

The continuous methodology is tied in with embracing change, not as a last objective but rather as a consistent cycle. It's a continuous obligation to live a better, more joyful life that you keep up with for as long as possible.

Celebrating Success: Reflecting on My Transformation

The journey of weight loss is often marked by milestones, challenges, and incredible transformations. But in our quest for change, it's crucial to pause and celebrate success. This chapter is a reflection on the profound transformation I've experienced and the importance of acknowledging and cherishing the journey.

The Significance of Celebrating Success

Celebrating success isn't just about a pat on the back or a momentary celebration; it's about acknowledging the immense effort and commitment that have gone into the journey. It's a reminder of the power of persistence and the incredible potential for change.

Reflecting on the Journey

As we delve into my transformation, I'll take you through the key moments and lessons that have shaped my path. These reflections are not just personal; they offer insights and inspiration for your own journey.

1. The Starting Point

Every transformation begins with a starting point. I'll share my own experiences and the factors that led me to take the first step toward change. It's a reminder that transformation often starts with a single decision.

2. The Early Challenges

The early days of any weight loss journey can be challenging. I'll recount my struggles, doubts, and the hurdles I faced. These experiences are a testament to the resilience needed to keep moving forward.

3. The Role of Support

Support plays a significant role in transformation. I'll share stories of the people who stood by me, offered encouragement, and helped me navigate the journey. It's a reminder that we don't have to go it alone.

4. Milestones and Achievements

Celebrating success is about acknowledging each milestone and achievement. I'll take you through the moments of triumph, the feeling of reaching goals, and the lessons learned along the way.

5. Setbacks and Resilience

No journey is without setbacks. I'll share my own experiences with setbacks and how they became stepping stones to greater resilience. Setbacks are not the end of the road; they're part of the journey.

6. The Transformation of Mindset

Transformation goes beyond physical changes; it's about a shift in mindset. I'll discuss how my perspective on health, food, and self-image has evolved throughout the journey.

7. Embracing New Habits

One of the keys to success is the development of new, sustainable habits. I'll share how I integrated healthier choices into my daily life and how these habits became second nature.

8. The Power of Patience

Patience is a virtue that cannot be overstated. I'll reflect on how patience became a guiding principle in my transformation and allowed me to navigate the ups and downs of the journey.

9. The Joy of Non-Scale Victories

Celebrating success isn't just about numbers on a scale. I'll discuss the importance of non-scale victories, from improved energy levels and better sleep to increased confidence and self-love.

10. Looking Ahead

Transformation is an ongoing process. I'll share my vision for the future and my commitment to maintaining the progress made. This chapter isn't an endpoint but a milestone on an ever-evolving journey.

Stories of Transformation

As we reflect on my transformation, we'll also hear stories of individuals who have undergone remarkable changes. These stories serve as a reminder that transformation is possible for anyone, regardless of their starting point.

The Importance of Your Journey

While my journey is a reflection of personal experiences, it's also an invitation for you to celebrate your own successes. Transformation is not confined to a single narrative; it's a collective experience shared by many on their unique paths to change.

Your Transformation Journey

As we delve into celebrating success and reflecting on transformation, I encourage you to consider your own journey. What successes have you achieved, and what transformations have you undergone? Celebrating success is not just about looking back; it's also about looking forward with determination and the knowledge that your journey continues.

CHAPTER 6

BONUS: MY RECIPE FOR SUCCESS

In the mission of enduring weight reduction and a better way of life, it frequently feels like we're looking for an enchanted recipe. Part 6 is an investigation of the recipe for progress that I've found through my excursion. It's anything but a mysterious equation, yet a mix of standards, propensities, and experiences have changed my life. This part is a challenge to find an interesting recipe for progress.

Elements for Progress

Achievement is a diverse idea. With regards to weight reduction, it's not just about numbers on a scale. It's a mix of actual wellbeing, mental prosperity, and general joy. How about we investigate the key fixings that make up my recipe for progress:

1. Mindset: The Establishment

Achievement begins with the right mentality. I'll dig into the significance of a positive and decided outlook in accomplishing your objectives. It's tied in with putting stock in yourself and your ability for change.

2. Objective Setting: The Guide

Clear and sensible objectives are like a guide for your journey. I'll examine the craft of setting significant, attainable targets and how they give guidance and inspiration.

3. Good dieting: The Fuel

Food is fuel for your body and psyche. I'll share my way to deal with good dieting, including the standards of adjusted sustenance, segment control, and careful eating.

4. Normal Activity: The Development

Practice is an imperative part of a solid way of life. I'll investigate the job of ordinary actual work in weight reduction and generally prosperity, including the significance of finding exercises you appreciate.

5. Consistency: The Paste

The fact that it binds the recipe makes consistency magic. I'll talk about how keeping up with consistency in your propensities, whether it's eating, working out, or taking care of oneself, is vital to making and supporting progress.

6. Resilience: The Security Net

Versatility is your security net when mishaps happen. I'll share techniques for creating profound flexibility and exploring difficulties with effortlessness.

7. Support: The Lift

Having an emotionally supportive network is a critical fix in progress. I'll investigate the different types of help, from loved ones to help gatherings and experts, and how they can lift you up.

8. Balance: The Agreement

Balance is vital to maintaining a solid way of life. I'll examine the significance of balance between fun and serious activities, a decent eating regimen, and tracking down harmony in your day to day daily schedule.

9. Self-Reflection: The Input

Self-reflection gives input to progress. I'll discuss the force of contemplation and how it assists you with gaining from your encounters and settling on better decisions.

10. Self-Compassion: The Consideration

Self-empathy is an essential fix. I'll make sense of how caring for yourself, even in snapshots of disappointment, is crucial for keeping up with inspiration and confidence.

11. Joy: The Zest of Life

Achievement ought to bring pleasure to your life. I'll investigate how tracking down bliss in your excursion, praising non-scale triumphs, and partaking in the process can fuel your inspiration.

12. Adaptability: The Adaptability

Life is erratic, and adaptability is fundamental. I'll talk about how adjusting to change and unexpected conditions is important for the recipe for progress.

Making an Exceptional Recipe

While my recipe for progress depends on my encounters and bits of knowledge, the magnificence of this part is the most ideal greeting for you to make your own extraordinary recipe. I'll direct you on the most proficient method to mix these fixings, changing the extents to suit your own excursion and objectives. Your recipe for progress is a customized mix that mirrors your qualities, wants, and goals.

Your Recipe for Progress

As we explore Chapter 6, I urge you to think about your own recipe for progress. What fixes do you have to accomplish your objectives? What standards reverberate with your remarkable excursion? Creating your recipe for progress isn't simply a hypothetical activity; it's a down to earth guide for changing your life.

Breakfast: How I Started My Day Right

Breakfast, when disregarded in my day to day daily practice, arose as a unique advantage in my weight reduction venture. At first, I accepted that skirting this dinner would speed up my advancement by decreasing my everyday calorie intake. Be that as it may, over time, I came to see the value in the vital role breakfast played in establishing the right vibe for my day and propelling my objectives.

The Meaning of Breakfast

Breakfast isn't known as the main dinner of the day without reason. This dinner, frequently dismissed or forfeited for the sake of time or caloric limitation, colossally affects our prosperity. The impetus gets your digestion into gear, offers fundamental supplements, and makes an establishment for your decisions over the course of the day.

1. Kicking off Your Digestion

Each day, when you have breakfast, you're successfully awakening your digestion. You're telling your body, "Now is the ideal time to get going." This implies that you'll consume calories all the more proficiently over the course of the day. In my excursion, I found that beginning the day with a healthy dinner was similar to firing up the motor, making way for better calorie consumption.

2. Forestalling Gorging Later

Skipping breakfast could appear to be a method for eliminating your day to day carbohydrate level, but it frequently misfires. At the point when you skirt this dinner, you're bound to end up starving by lunch or bite time. The outcome? Unfortunate food decisions and bigger parts Breakfast, I found, was the way to holding my hunger in line and forestalling those late morning gorges.

3. Giving Fundamental Supplements

Breakfast conveys indispensable supplements to your body. It's an excellent chance to support yourself with nutrients, minerals, protein, and fiber. A nutritious breakfast gives you the energy and food you need to handle your day. Missing breakfast implied I was passing up these fundamental supplements.

4. Supporting Solid Decisions

Beginning your day with a solid breakfast establishes an inspirational vibe for your dietary decisions. Having a decent breakfast made me bound to pursue better choices over the course of the day. It turned into my anchor, directing me towards better decisions.

5. Supporting Mental Capability

Breakfast isn't just about sustaining your body; it's essential for your mind's exhibition. A healthy morning feast worked on my fixation, sharpness, and by and large mental capacities. It resembles giving fuel to your mind, making it daily where you're terminating on all chambers.

6. Making Routine and Construction

Fostering a morning meal routine offered me a feeling of construction and consistency in my day to day existence. It was a method for beginning every day with expectation, building up my obligation to a better way of life. Rather than heedlessly snatching something in a hurry or selecting the comfort of an energized drink, breakfast brought discipline and construction into my mornings.

My Morning Meal Change

As I integrated breakfast into my everyday daily schedule, I discovered that it was not just about eating something toward the beginning of the day; it was tied in with consuming a sound and adjusted feast. This is the way I changed my morning meal propensities:

1. Adjusting Macronutrients

An effective breakfast incorporates an equilibrium of starches, protein, and healthy fats. My decisions frequently include an entire grain toast with avocado and eggs or a bowl of cereal with nuts and berries. This mix provided support and energy over the course of the morning.

2. Keeping away from Sweet Cereals and Cakes

Sweet grains and baked goods, albeit helpful, weren't the most ideal choices for a nutritious breakfast. I avoided these less solid decisions and zeroed in on entire food sources.

3. Focusing on Protein

Protein was the foundation of my morning meal schedule. It helped me feel full and fulfilled, diminishing the desire to nibble on less sound choices later in the day. I frequently consolidated wellsprings of protein, for example, Greek yogurt, curds, or lean meats.

4. Consolidating Fiber

Fiber was one more fundamental part of my morning meal. It helped with processing and added to a sensation of completion. Organic products, vegetables, and entire grains were my go-to sources of fiber.

5. Remaining Hydrated

Hydration was important for my wake-up routine. I'd begin the day with a glass of water, which assisted with hydration as well as aided in controlling my hunger.

6. Dinner Arranging

To guarantee I had sound breakfast choices promptly accessible, I integrated dinner planning into my everyday practice. This assisted me in trying not to go after less nutritious decisions on occupied mornings.

The Advantages of a Solid Breakfast

Integrating a nutritious breakfast into my day to day schedule brought a few benefits:

1. Supported Energy

A healthy breakfast gave me the energy I expected to start my day with essentialness. I was not languid at this point in the first part of the day, and I felt prepared to handle my day to day errands.

2. Craving Control

Breakfast held my craving under control, diminishing the probability of eating on less sound choices. It gave me a feeling of completion that endured throughout the day.

3. Better Food Decisions

With breakfast establishing an uplifting vibe, I found it more straightforward to pursue better food decisions over the course of the day. Maybe a solid breakfast gave an establishment to careful eating.

4. Further developed Fixation

Mental execution and fixation improved fundamentally. I was more ready and centered, making me more useful at work and in different parts of my life.

5. Weight reduction and Support

Consolidating a solid breakfast played a vital part in my weight reduction and upkeep venture. It helped me accomplish and keep a sound load by launching my digestion and advancing adjusted dietary patterns. Skipping breakfast was presently not a choice; it had turned into the foundation of my everyday practice, directing me towards a better and more seriously satisfying way of life. Breakfast was my mysterious element for beginning every day on the right note.

Lunch: Finding Balance In The Midday Meal

Lunch, frequently sandwiched between the hurrying around of our regular routines, holds a one of a kind spot in the excursion of weight reduction and a better way of life. It's an amazing chance to refuel our bodies, sustain our psyches, and track down the equilibrium that keeps us on target. In this section, I'll share how I tracked down harmony in the late morning feast, making it a necessary piece of my recipe for progress.

The Early afternoon Challenge

For some, lunch can be a difficult feast. It's when occupied plans, work responsibilities, and individual obligations unite. Previously, I frequently wound up settling on rushed food decisions, forfeiting nourishment for comfort. Notwithstanding, the late morning feast's significance before long became obvious.

1. An Increase in Energy

Lunch isn't simply a feast; a wellspring of energy brings you through the rest of your day. An even lunch can assist with combating the midday downturn and keep you useful and centered.

2. Hunger Control

A wonderful lunch keeps up with hunger control, decreasing the possibilities that arise during the later part of the day. I saw that when I dismissed lunch or settled on unfortunate decisions, I was bound to nibble on undesirable choices.

3. Supplement Top off

Your body's supplement repositories can become exhausted by noontime. Lunch is a chance to recharge fundamental nutrients, minerals, and different supplements, guaranteeing your body has what it needs to ideally work.

4. Keeping up with Digestion

Consuming a decent lunch maintains consistent digestion, empowering your body to productively consume calories and maintain a healthy weight.

5. Mental Clarity

Lunch feeds the body as well as supports mental lucidity and sharpness. It's fuel for the cerebrum, empowering you to use wise judgment and stay zeroed in on errands.

6. Profound Prosperity

The late morning dinner isn't just about actual wellbeing; it's an opportunity to have some time off and partake in a snapshot of unwinding. This break can definitely affect your profound prosperity by diminishing pressure and advancing equilibrium in your day.

Tracking down Equilibrium in My Lunch

As I set out on my weight reduction venture, I understood the significance of tracking down balance in my lunch. I changed this feast into a conscious decision as opposed to a hurried choice. This is the way I achieved equilibrium:

1. Focusing on Entire Food varieties

A decent lunch includes entire food varieties rich in supplements. I zeroed in on consolidating various vegetables, lean proteins, entire grains, and sound fats into my early afternoon dinner. This approach fulfilled my dietary requirements as well as gave me a feeling of totality.

2. Keeping away from Cheap Food Traps

Hurrying through lunch frequently prompts snatching cheap food or accommodation things. I put forth a cognizant attempt to avoid these less nutritious decisions. This choice upheld my wellbeing as well as emphatically affected my energy levels.

3. Careful Eating

Lunch wasn't simply a dinner to consume; it turned into a chance for careful eating. I took as much time as is needed to relish each nibble, perceiving the flavors and surfaces of my food. This care permitted me to check out my body's yearning and completion signs.

4. Appropriate Hydration

I integrated legitimate hydration into my lunch routine by having a glass of water or natural tea with my dinner. This upheld my hydration as well as assisted with hunger control.

5. Feast Arranging

Similarly, as I executed the feast anticipating breakfast, I stretched out this training to lunch. Planning snacks ahead of time saved time as well as guaranteed that I had nutritious and adjusted dinners promptly accessible.

The Advantages of a Reasonable Lunch

Integrating a reasonable lunch into my everyday schedule brought a few critical advantages:

1. Practical Energy

An even lunch gave the energy expected to ride out the day. It implied that I was not really feeling depleted or drowsy in the early evening.

2. Craving Control

Lunch kept up with my craving control, lessening the possibility of careless nibbling or gorging later in the day.

3. Nourishing Top off

Recharging fundamental supplements during lunch emphatically affected my general prosperity. I felt more sustained and better, both actually and intellectually.

4. Keeping up with Digestion

A reasonable lunch kept my digestion on target, making it more effective at consuming calories and aiding weight loss.

5. Mental Clarity

The right noontime feast guaranteed that I stayed ready and centered in the early evening, making me more useful in my work and day to day assignments.

6. Close to home Prosperity

Finding the opportunity to partake in a fair lunch made snapshots of unwinding in my day. It gave a valuable chance to destress and track down close to home equilibrium.

The Mission for Noontime Equilibrium

Lunch changed from a rushed need to a careful and feeding feast. It turned into a snapshot of equilibrium in my day, a cognizant decision that upheld my wellbeing and prosperity. Finding balance in the noontime feast was one more move toward my excursion towards a better and more joyful life.

Dinner: The Delightful End to My Day

Supper, the last venture of my day to day culinary excursion, is a loved and significant dinner. It's the second time I can loosen up, enjoy a fantastic dinner, and ponder the day. In this section, I'll share how I've come to see supper as an awesome finish to my day.

The Night Hour

Supper means the change from the hecticness of the day to a more loose and quiet night. It's a chance to slow down, partake in the organization of friends and family, and sustain both body and soul. Supper holds a unique spot in my heart as the night unfurls.

1. Association and Holding

Supper frequently turns into a mutual undertaking in the night, a second for families and companions to meet up, share stories, and reconnect. The feeling of fellowship and holding that supper encourages is a wellspring of delight and close to home sustenance.

2. Culinary Innovativeness

Evening suppers take into account culinary innovativeness. It's the second time I can investigate new recipes, explore different avenues regarding flavors, and savor the experience of the demonstration of cooking. The most common way of getting ready for supper is essentially as compensating as partaking in the actual feast.

3. Careful Eating

In the calm of the night, I've figured out how to embrace being careful during supper. I enjoy each nibble, appreciate the surfaces and flavors, and pay attention to my body's signs of completion. This training makes supper wonderful as well as advances a feeling of equilibrium.

4. Sustenance and Recuperation

Supper gives sustenance, recharging the supplements consumed over the course of the day. It upholds recuperation and restoration, guaranteeing that I get up the following day feeling revived and prepared for another day.

5. Pondering the Day

As I plunk down for supper, I frequently ponder the day's achievements and difficulties. It's a snapshot of appreciation, a chance to celebrate accomplishments and gain from difficulties. Supper fills in as the ideal setting for consideration and mindfulness.

Difficult exercise in Supper

While supper is a period for unwinding and happiness, it likewise presents a valuable chance to keep up with the equilibrium I've developed over the course of the day. This is the way I've accomplished this balance in my nightly dinner:

1. Adjusted Supplements

Supper, as with other feasts, is a fair creation of supplements. I consolidate vegetables, lean proteins, entire grains, and healthy fats into my nightly dinner. This equilibrium guarantees I get the essential sustenance to fuel my body and support my general prosperity.

2. Segment Control

Controlling piece sizes is fundamental during supper. It prevents gorging, advances absorption, and guarantees that I awaken feeling good as opposed to excessively full.

3. Slow and Careful Feasting

I've embraced a sluggish and careful way to deal with supper. This includes eating at a comfortable speed, partaking in the feast, and being completely present during supper. A demonstration of taking care of oneself improves my overall experience.

4. Hydration

Remaining hydrated is urgent at supper. I polish off a glass of water or home grown tea to help process and keep me hydrated.

5. Light Night Tidbits

In the event that I feel the need for a nibble at night, I settle on light and nutritious decisions like a natural product or yogurt. These choices check desires without over-burdening my framework before sleep time.

The Joys of Supper

Supper, the superb finish to my day, holds a mother lode of joys. It's a snapshot of association, culinary investigation, and reflection. It offers the ideal chance to offset sustenance with unwinding, encouraging a feeling of prosperity and happiness as I plan to embrace the evening.

CONCLUSION

EMBRACING A HEALTHIER LIFE

As we finish up this journey, the acknowledgment turns out to be clear: the quest for a better life isn't simply an objective; it's a long lasting odyssey. It's an excursion set apart by change, misfortunes, and, most importantly, versatility.

We've investigated the meaning of breakfast, the late morning equilibrium of lunch, and the great finish to the day at supper. Every dinner, a structure block of our day to day presence, has turned into a material for making a better and more joyful life.

Yet, this journey isn't bound to the domain of dinners alone. It's tied in with developing a positive outlook, tracking down bliss in development, embracing support, and valuing each triumph—of all shapes and sizes.

Embracing a better human existence is much more than flawlessness; it's about progress. It's a pledge to change, a guarantee to oneself to continue to push ahead, to get ourselves when we stagger, and to praise each bit closer to our desires.

The way to a better life is remarkable for every one of us. It's anything but an unbending equation; however, it's a customized recipe—a mix of nourishment, action, care, and self-empathy.

Thus, as we finish up this excursion, we should recall that the way to a better life is definitely not a limited course; it's a continuous experience. It's a day to day existence improved by our decisions, the illustrations we learn, and the delight we track down in each second. Embrace it, for it's the most beneficial excursion you'll at any point embrace.

Here's to a better life where every day is an open door and every feast is an opportunity to enjoy the delight of residing great.

www.ingramcontent.com/pod-product-compliance
Lightning Source LLC
Chambersburg PA
CBHW050853260726
48660CB00006B/2606